The Mediterranean Diet Cookbook

The Complete Mediterranean Diet Meal Prep Guide For Healthy Lifestyle And Weight Loss

(4 Weeks Of Recipes & Meal Plans To Lose Weight)

Sara Shirley

Published by Jason Thawne Publishing House

© Sara Shirley

The Mediterranean Diet Cookbook: The Complete Mediterranean Diet Meal Prep Guide For Healthy Lifestyle And Weight Loss
(4 Weeks of Recipes & Meal Plans To Lose Weight)

All Rights Reserved

ISBN   978-1-989749-83-8

This document is geared towards providing exact and reliable information in regards to the topic and issue covered. The publication is sold with the idea that the publisher isn't required to render accounting, officially permitted, or otherwise, qualified services. If advice is necessary, legal or even professional, a practiced individual in the profession should be ordered.

- From a Declaration of Principles which was accepted and approved equally by a Committee of the American Bar Association and a Committee of Publishers and Associations.

In no way is it legal to reproduce, duplicate, or even transmit any part of this document in either electronic means or in printed format. Recording of this publication is strictly prohibited and any storage of this document isn't allowed unless with proper written permission from the publisher. All rights reserved.

The information provided herein is stated to be truthful and consistent, in that any liability, in terms of inattention or otherwise, by any usage or abuse of any policies, processes, or directions contained within is the solitary and also utter responsibility of the recipient reader. Under no circumstances will any legal responsibility or blame be held against the publisher for any reparation, damages, or monetary loss due to the information herein, either directly or indirectly.

Respective authors own all copyrights not held by the publisher.

The information herein is offered for just informational purposes solely, and is universal as so. The presentation of the information is without contract or any type of guarantee assurance.

The trademarks that are used are without any consent, and also the publication of the trademark is without permission or backing by the trademark owner. All trademarks and brands within this book are for clarifying purposes only and are the owned by the owners themselves, not affiliated with this document.

TABLE OF CONTENTS

PART 1 1

INTRODUCTION 2

CHAPTER 1: WHAT IS THE MEDITERRANEAN DIET? 6

CHAPTER 2: WHAT'S DOES THE MEDITERRANEAN DIET CONSIST OF? 12

HIGH AMOUNT OF PLANT FOODS 12
INTERESTING AND DIFFERENT DESSERT 13
HIGH ON BEANS 13
OLIVE OIL 13
DAIRY 14
MODERATE FISH AND FEWER EGGS 14
REDUCED RED MEAT 14
WINE 15
FATS 15
LEGUMES 15

CHAPTER 3: BENEFITS OF THE MEDITERRANEAN DIET 17

CHAPTER 4: FIVE LIPSMACKING RECIPES 25

ROASTED VEGETABLES WITH POLENTA 25

SPANISH CAULIFLOWER RICE: 27
GREEK FAVA: 28
KUMQUAT TAGINE (MOROCCAN STEW) 31
GREEK BREAKFAST FRITTATA: 32

CONCLUSION: 34

PART 2 36

INTRODUCTION	37
BAD FATS	58
LEARNING TO READ LABELS	63
CONCLUSION	96
ABOUT THE AUTHOR	96

Part 1

Introduction

As soon as the alarm goes off, the race towards that invisible finish line begins! We begin darting through the day, hardly pausing to catch a breath, let alone a healthy meal. We try to keep the energy levels up by grabbing convenient foods like burgers, pizzas, soda and whatnot. While caught up in work, we hardly pay attention to the flavors in the food that we eat, let alone the nutrients present in it.

We become conscious of what we eat only when we hit rock bottom- when we become obese! Obesity equates to diabetes, cardiac issues and a plethora of diseases that follow suit. When we realize the need to correct our dietary habits, we find ourselves as a part of a new race! The race behind that perfect diet plan that will help you lose pounds in a jiffy.

Needless to say, there are several kinds of diets out there, some very restrictive and some quite liberal. We end up trying everything under the sun and give up midway because we find it difficult to eliminate certain kinds of foodstuffs all of a sudden. Every diet expects us to say no to those mouth watering desserts or meat products or exquisite seafood. It is human tendency to crave for those things that are forbidden to us. So is the case with food and that is the reason why most of us fail while trying to follow these diets.

Just like how there is an exception to the general rule, there exists a diet that is not restrictive in nature but still benefits you in ways more than those fancy restrictive diets! This exceptional yet effective diet is known as the Mediterranean diet. The Mediterranean diet was discovered as early as 1900s when medical research proved that people who resided in the Eastern Mediterranean regions lived a healthier and longer life as compared to the people who lived in the other parts of the world.

What is so special about the Mediterranean diet? The Mediterranean diet is all about consuming different ingredients in different proportions. It is built in such a way that the risks associated with certain kinds of foodstuffs like red meat or dairy products is negated by the inclusion of fresh vegetables, fruits and nuts. You can still have your red meat, but not in the same quantum and frequency as your fish. Yes, the Mediterranean diet is all about striking that perfect balance among all kinds of foodstuffs.

You can not only reduce those extra pounds but also reduce the risks of several chronic diseases like Alzheimer's, Parkinson's, diabetes, stroke and several cardiovascular diseases. Following this diet also regulates the rate of metabolism of your body and keeps you active throughout the day. Say yes to increased longevity with this diet.

In this e-book, we bring to you several exciting recipes that are delicious as well as healthy! Go on and try them! You will not be disappointed. Follow this diet and be physically active to experience the change in your body. Thank you for downloading this eBook.

Chapter 1: What Is The Mediterranean diet?

In this first chapter we will take a broad look about what the Mediterranean Diet is all about and how it can affect your body.

As explained in the introduction the Mediterranean diet was in a way discovered in the 1900s by observing the diet of the non English speaking regions of Europe. It was found that the people living in Eastern Mediterranean regions were living a healthy and quite long life as compared to their English speaking comrades. This the researchers realized was happening because of their diet which was and is quite healthy and fresh as compared to the traditional English or Anglo-Saxon diet.

It is believed that we can classify the Western European diets into two categories, the Northern European diet and the Southern European diet. The Mediterranean diet is considered to be a south European diet. It is highly focused on the diet and food habits of people of Southern Italy, Crete and large portion of Greece. Nowadays even Spain, Portugal and Southern France are included in the list even though there is no Mediterranean coast in Portugal. It is seen that people living in these nations are lean, fit, and healthy and look really attractive. So what in the name of Food God does their food and diet contains or why is it so effective?

Mediterranean diet is so effective as well as popular because it not restrictive. It is all about eating different things in different proportions. This means you can eat everything except that the proportions will be changed. Interesting huh? You can eat a lot of things but if they are not mentioned in your diet then you will have to eat very less proportions of it. For instance if you are a great fan of red meat, which incidentally is not eaten in large proportion in Mediterranean diet, you can eat it but in less proportion, instead you should eat high amounts of vegetables, fresh fruits as well as nuts. You will still be able to eat red meat no doubt just in fewer amounts.

It is all about making an interesting combination of various foods and food items and Mediterranean diet is a useful and interesting combination of fresh food as well as cooked food thus making it one of the best diets.

As we said earlier that the Mediterranean diets became really popular in the 1990s which was quite heavily publicized by De Ancel Keys who made it popular in the 1990s when he was stationed in Italy. When he made it famous people were quite perplexed about it. Diets are always believed to be something which can only cause harm and nothing else. You are supposed to stay hungry all the time on a diet and you cannot enjoy anything of your choice because it will be against your diet. All of these and many more are the reasons why diets although being popular are looked down upon. This is why when Mediterranean diet became popular in the 1990s people got confused. You do not need to starve yourself on Mediterranean diet. You eat whatever you want albeit in right proportions.

The diet when it became popular also confused researchers as it is considered to be very high in fats. Although fat consumption is high in this diet yet the prevalence of diseases and disorders such as cardiovascular diseases, hypertension, obesity, cancer, diabetes etc is very low in the nations mention above as compared to the northern European nations and USA.

It is no surprise that USA is being mentioned with Northern European nations here because the diet of the USA is very much similar to that of the nations of the Northern Europe. This northern European and USA diet consists of high amounts of red meat, butter as well as animal fats, and low amounts of vegetables, fresh fruits etc. In comparison the nations of the Southern Europe such as Italy, Spain, Greece and France have diet which is quite rich in fruits and vegetables as well as good quality fats.

Even other nations such as Belgium, Netherlands, Germany, Austria, Switzerland etc of the northern Europe have very well adopted the Mediterranean diet whereas the nations such as UK, Ireland and other nations like USA, Australia, New Zealand etc still have not. Notice a thing here; the nations which have adopted the Mediterranean diet are non-English speaking nations. Some researchers believe that this is the reason why people from non English speaking nations have a long and healthy life as compared with the English speaking nations.

It is also believed that the amount and the type of the beverage which is drunk frequently in these nations have big effect on the lifestyle as well as obesity. The Mediterranean people consume high amounts of red wine while in comparison the nations of the Northern Europe as well as USA consume large amounts of beer.

Red wine is considered to be healthier as compared to beer as red wine contains flavonoids. These flavonoids are quite powerful antioxidants which are highly useful for human body.

It is also believed that one of the major reasons why the Mediterranean diet is more popular and healthy Anglo-Saxon diet because it contains high amounts of raw and unprocessed food. This is considered to be one of the best reasons why a person should adopt a Mediterranean diet

Chapter 2: What's Does The Mediterranean Diet Consist Of?

In the previous chapter we discussed some basic details about the Mediterranean diet while in this chapter we will focus on what exactly goes into a Mediterranean diet. We will look at the various things which are quite popular and eaten often in a Mediterranean diet one by one in detail now.

High Amount of Plant Foods

One of the major reasons why this Mediterranean diet is so popular is because of the high amounts of plant derived foods which you need to eat while being on this diet. These sources are varied and you may eat leaves, fruits, stems, roots, and even flowers. These plant sources and plant derived products are most of the times consumed while they are still fresh thus making them even more healthy.

Interesting and Different Dessert

You must be thinking that I am pulling your leg. A dessert on a diet! But don't worry it is perfectly true. Mediterranean diet promotes eating dessert because majority of their deserts are actually fresh fruits. Fresh suits can be also frozen and then served to create an interesting dessert.

High on Beans

Mediterranean diet is rich in food items such as cereals, nuts and beans. The cereals such as oats, wheat, brown rice, and corn are very much popular in the Mediterranean diet. All of these if eaten in proportion are quite healthy and can provided body with the energy it is suppose dot have.

Olive Oil

No we are not talking about Popeye's girlfriend we are talking about the oil. Olive oil of various kinds is used all over the Mediterranean coast and the regions where Mediterranean diet is popular.

Olive oil is a very good source of healthy fats.

Dairy

The Mediterranean diet consists of high amounts of dairy products such as cheese and yogurt. These are also good source of good fats and proteins.

Moderate Fish and Fewer Eggs

Mediterranean diet is more concentrated upon vegetables as compared to meat and eggs. It is advised that people eat fish in moderation while on a Mediterranean diet and that they should not eat more than four eggs per week.

Reduced Red Meat

If re meat is your favorite kind of meat you will have to adjust a lot because red meat is nearly prohibited from this diet. Very less amounts of red meat is allowed every week. As compared to the Northern European diet, the amount of red meat allowed in Mediterranean diet is almost negligible.

Wine

As explained earlier, the Mediterranean diet consist more of wine. People also love to drink wine as compared to the American or English who prefer beer. As explained earlier wine contains flavonoides which are quite essential for the body.

Fats

The Mediterranean diet consists of high amounts of good quality fats. These fats .i.e. monosaturated fats are present in high numbers as compared to the saturated fats in Mediterranean diet. This diet because of its high amounts of raw food is also quite rich in fiber.

Legumes

Mediterranean diet consists of high amounts of legumes like the Indian diet. Legumes are basically seeds of various plants such as peas, chick peas, alfalfa, beans etc. These are rich sources of protein and other vital nutrients and thus form an important part of the Mediterranean diet. Legumes are also responsible for improving the glycemic control of the patients of type 2 diabetes. They are also supposed to reduce the risk of coronary heart disease.

So far in this chapter we have covered what are the major components of Mediterranean diet. In the next chapter let's look at what are the major benefits of adopting a Mediterranean diet.

Chapter 3: Benefits of the Mediterranean Diet

So far we have talked about the various components and food items present in the Mediterranean diet and have also looked at the basics of a Mediterranean diet. In this chapter we will look at the various benefits associated with a Mediterranean diet and also why you should adopt it for becoming a fit, healthy and active person.

Mediterranean diet has a lot of benefits which are extremely varied. Some of the main benefits have been found because of extensive and sophisticated research which has made Mediterranean diet popular all over the world. Most of these results were achieved by comparing the two popular diets the Northern European diet/ USA diet and the Mediterranean diet. Now let us look at the various benefits of Mediterranean diet.

According to an article publish in October 2012 on Food Technolofy3 it was explained how diets which are high on plant sources can actually reduce or even totally eliminate the chances of developing chronic diseases for instance cardiovascular diseases, type 2 diabetes, cancer etc. The Mediterranean diet is also supposed to reduce the risk of stroke and various other such genetic disorders which can even cause deaths. This it can be said that Mediterranean diet is a superhero which can save lives.

In BMJ Open 5 an Italian study was published which put forward the theory saying that people following a Mediterranean diet have a high quality life and also have better health-related quality life- HRQL. They also proposed that the Mediterranean diet is also very much good for the mental health. It contains many nutrients which are quite good for the brain as well as the body.

A study published in the Archives of Internal Medicine by the McMaster university have proposed that any diet consisting certain food groups and dietary nutrients such as nuts, monosaturated fats, vegetables, fruits etc i.e. everything which is considered to be 'healthy' is very good for your heart. As you can clearly see that this description clearly fits the Mediterranean diet thus Mediterranean diet is highly good for your heart and blood supply. It will help you to keep your heart healthy and strong. It is also good for your circulatory system and as it not high in cholesterol it will also prevent clogs.

According to a study released by the BMJ it is proposed that the Mediterranean diet in its traditional form can actually prevent the onset of type 2 diabetes in an individual. It can thus protect people from diabetes. Of course you will also have to accompany the diet with exercise if you want the complete benefits.

According to another research the Mediterranean diet is very much good for your brain too. As said earlier it is quite good for your mental health but it is also good for the overall wellbeing of the brain. It is said to reduce the damage caused to the little blood vessels present in the brain. These findings were published in the Archives of Neurology.

A study was published in the JCEM I.e. the Journal of Clinical Endocrinology and Metabolism which has proposed that the high amounts of olive oil present in the Mediterranean diet increases the amount of osteocalin in body which in turn is highly effective in protection of bones. It is especially important in children as well as elderly whose bones are weaker as compared to that of the young people. Olive oil is used in various preparations in Mediterranean diet and thus one can get enough amount of osteocalin through the Mediterranean diet.

A highly researched study published in the American Journal of Medicine has proposed that the people who have adopted or have been adopting Mediterranean diet as their diet have reduced their risk of heart diseases and heart attack. This risk is even lower than the people who follow a strict low-fat diet thus debunking the age old myth that not all fat is bad for your body. A said earlier that this diet contains a lot of olive oil which is a rich source of monosaturated fatty acids that is highly effective against cholesterol.

Another interesting study has proposed that a Mediterranean diet can also slow the aging process. The large amounts of olive old, fresh fruits, vegetables, nuts as well as the red wine with meal are supposed to reduce the signs of aging. Especially the high amounts of olive oil present in the Mediterranean diet is said to be a really good anti-aging agent which can even reduce wrinkles, crows feet etc and can act as a skin tightening agent. It has been used since the ancient times to as a beauty product and a cosmetic and is thus a proven product to enhance your looks. The diet is also supposed to give you good hair nails, reduce hair fall, clear skin blemishes and give you an overall fresh look and glowing skin.

The diet is also supposed to prevent Alzheimer's disease and Parkinson's disease as well. The diet is a great way to regulate your metabolism and bodily functions. It is really good for your digestion and you will probably never suffer from IBS after starting this diet due to its fiber rich components. As the diet contains high amounts of fresh fruits and vegetables it is supposed to make your body feels light and active. You will feel a constant energy force running through your body and fatigue will stay away from you. You will be able to do lots of work without getting tired easily.

The major reason why anyone should adopt this diet is that it can be used to counter obesity effectively. If you are obese, overweight or are worried about getting overweight this diet can prove to be a boon for you. You can easily achieve your target weight or can keep on your current weight by adopting this diet and a suitable exercise plan. This diet alone can also be used to reduce weight and fats but it is always better to accompany it with a proper exercise plan which will increase the speed of the weight loss. As the Mediterranean diet is not a fad diet or anything like that this diet has relatively no side effects. Although you might feel withdrawal symptoms if you are absolutely in love with red meat at first but once you start making and eating the recipes mentioned in this eBook you will definitely forget about the red meat. This diet is highly effective in weight loss as it promotes the burning of the already present body fat and also prevents its accumulation. As it is actually a kind of a lifestyle and not a fad diet the weight lost with the help of this diet will not be a short term loss but will be a long term or even permanent loss. This diet is suitable for anyone and everyone including kids, teens, adults, elders etc again because it is a lifestyle option and not a fad diet. But still it might be important to check with your physician before starting this diet.

A very important aspect of this diet is that it can be adopted by almost anyone so even if you are a vegan or a vegetarian person or are lactose intolerant or are bound by religion to eat only certain things, you need not to worry, you can find good recipes online and in this book which will let you follow this diet without forgoing any other commitment. This diet is thus very adjustable and can be adapted according to each person's personal choices and tastes. So if you don't eat pork, or milk, or nuts etc you need not to worry, just follow some recipes which avoid these things and you are good to go.

Chapter 4: Five Lipsmacking Recipes

Roasted Vegetables with Polenta

Ingredients:

- 2 small butternut squashes, peeled, cut into 2 centimeter cubes
- 400 g beetroot, peeled , cut into 2 centimeter cubes
- 4 small red onions, cut into thin wedges
- 6 tablespoons olive oil
- Juice of a lemon
- 400 g fine polenta
- Black pepper powder to taste
- ¼ teaspoon white pepper powder
- 2 liters water
- 1 teaspoon salt
- 100 g butter
- 50 g parmesan cheese
- 50 g taleggio cheese
- Few rocket lettuce leaves to serve
- 2 tablespoons fresh thyme leaves

For the parmesan crisps:

- 100 g parmesan, grated

Method:

1. To make the parmesan crisps: Place the parmesan over a greased baking tray. Sprinkle black pepper powder over it. Bake in a preheated oven at 350 degree F for 5 minutes until light golden color.
2. Cool for a while. Break the parmesan into pieces using your fingers.
3. Place the squash and beetroot in a baking tin. Sprinkle oil, salt, pepper and lemon juice. Toss well.
4. Bake at 375 degree F for about 20 minutes. Add the onion wedges, mix well and bake for another 20-25 minutes or until cooked.
5. Boil the water with salt. Add half the butter. Slowly add the polenta, stirring constantly. Lower heat and simmer for about 30-35 minutes. Stir on and off. When cooked, the polenta should be thick and soft. If it is too dry, then add more water.
6. When cooked, add rest of the butter, parmesan, taleggio, and white pepper

powder. Mix well and remove from heat.
7. Serve the cooked polenta on individual plates. Sprinkle the roasted vegetables along with its juices. Sprinkle the parmesan crisps. Spread the rocket leaves over
8. The vegetables and crisps and finally top with thyme. Serve immediately

Spanish Cauliflower Rice:

Ingredients:
- 2 heads cauliflower, grated
- 8 cloves garlic, chopped
- 2 green bell peppers, chopped
- 2 red bell peppers, chopped
- 4 stalks celery chopped
- 4 small zucchinis, chopped
- ¼ cup oil
- 1 cup vegetable broth or stock
- 12 ounce tomato paste
- 2 tablespoons ground cumin
- 2 tablespoons dried oregano
- 1 teaspoon red chilli flakes or to taste

- 1 teaspoon salt or to taste
- 2 teaspoons lemon pepper

Method:

1. Place a skillet over medium heat. Add oil. When the oil heats up, add onions, garlic, pepper, zucchini, celery and cauliflower. Sauté for 3-4 minutes.
2. Lower heat. Add stock. Stir on and off.
3. When the cauliflower is slightly soft, add the tomato paste, cumin, oregano, red chilli flakes, salt, and lemon pepper. Mix well. Cook until the cauliflower has the consistency of cooked rice. If the cauliflower is too dry and not yet cooked, then add some more broth.
4. Add more seasonings if you desire. Serve hot with sausages.

Greek Fava:

Ingredients:

- 1 ½ cups yellow split peas, picked, rinsed, soaked in water for 30 minutes
- 6 tablespoons extra virgin olive oil, divided

- 1 large red onion, finely chopped
- 4 cups vegetable broth or water and extra if necessary
- 24 ounce squid or calamari, fresh or frozen, cleaned, cut into ½ inch rings, leave the tentacles on
- 1 ½ teaspoon salt, divided
- ½ teaspoon freshly ground pepper powder or to taste
- ¼ cup lemon juice
- 4 tablespoons fresh parsley, finely chopped
- Few lemon wedges

Method:

1. Place a saucepan over medium heat. Add 2 tablespoons oil. When oil is heated, add onions and sauté until translucent.
2. Add split peas and sauté for about 2 minutes. Add broth or water and bring to a boil.
3. When it starts boiling, cover, lower heat and simmer.
4. Cook until the split peas are tender. It takes about an hour to cook. If the

liquid has dried up, then add some more broth or water. When the split peas are cooked, remove from heat and keep aside for a little while to cool.
5. Meanwhile, mix together the squid rings, tentacles, 1 tablespoon oil, 1 teaspoon salt, and pepper. Keep aside for a while.
6. When cool enough to handle, transfer the peas to the food processor along with 1 tablespoon oil, lemon juice, and ½ teaspoon salt. Blend until smooth.
7. Transfer the blended split peas onto a serving platter and keep aside.
8. Fix the squid and tentacles onto skewers. Grease the grill rack. Place the skewers with the squids in a preheated grill and grill on medium high for about 4 minutes. Turn the skewer once.
9. When done, remove the squid and tentacles and lay over the split peas. Sprinkle the remaining olive oil, parsley, a little salt and pepper. Serve with lemon wedges

Kumquat Tagine (Moroccan Stew)

Ingredients:
- ½ tablespoon extra virgin olive oil
- 1 onion, thinly sliced
- 4 cloves garlic, slivered
- ½ tablespoon fresh ginger, minced
- 1 pound chicken thighs, skinless, boneless, trimmed of fat, cut into 2 inch pieces
- 1 teaspoon ground coriander
- 1 teaspoon ground cumin
- ½ teaspoon ground cinnamon
- Salt to taste
- Pepper powder to taste
- A large pinch powdered cloves
- 7 ounce vegetable broth
- 6 ounce kumquats, seeded, chopped
- ½ a 15 ounce can chickpeas, rinsed
- ¾ tablespoon honey

Method:
1. Pour oil in an oven proof casserole. Place over medium heat. Add onions, sauté until translucent. Add garlic and

ginger and sauté for a minute more. Keep stirring.
2. Add chicken and sauté for 7-8 minutes. Add ground coriander, cumin, and cinnamon. Also add salt, pepper, and cloves. Sauté for a few seconds until fragrant.
3. Add broth, kumquats, chickpeas, and honey. Simmer for a while.
4. Transfer the casserole into the preheated oven. Cover and bake at 375 degree F for about an hour.
5. Serve hot.

Greek Breakfast Frittata:

Ingredients:

- ½ a 14.5 ounce diced tomatoes, drained
- 1 small zucchini, cut into ½ inch pieces
- ½ tablespoons olive oil
- 2 cloves garlic, mined
- ¼ teaspoon dried basil
- ¼ teaspoon dried oregano
- ½ teaspoon Spike seasoning or any seasoning of your choice

- Freshly ground black pepper to taste
- 3 eggs, beaten
- ½ tablespoon milk
- ¼ cup mozzarella, grated
- 2 tablespoons feta cheese, grated

Method:

1. Place a heavy bottomed frying pan (that can be placed under the broiler) over medium heat.
2. Add olive oil to it. When the oil is heated, add zucchini, garlic, pepper powder, spike seasoning, oregano, and basil. Sauté for 3-4 minutes.
3. Add tomatoes and sauté until the moisture in the tomatoes is nearly dried up.
4. Meanwhile, add milk to the beaten eggs. Whisk well. Pour this mixture into the pan over the zucchini-tomato mixture. Do not stir until the eggs are just beginning to set.
5. Add half the mozzarella and feta. Now mix gently and let it cook for 2-3 minutes.

6. Now sprinkle the remaining half mozzarella and feta all over. Cover the pan and cook until the cheese melts.
7. Transfer the pan under a preheated broiler. Broil until light golden brown.
8. When done, let it cool slightly. Slice into wedges and serve immediately.

Conclusion:

Wasn't it refreshing to know that there exists a diet plan that didn't expect you to let go of certain kinds of foodstuffs yet serve the purpose? As you might have noticed from the recipes, the Mediterranean diet is not made up of boring green smoothies or bland soups.

On the other hand, they are rich in flavors as well as nutrients. Hence the Mediterranean diet serves twin purposes – satisfying your palette as well as taking care of your health! Well, you could not have asked for more!

Well, now that you know what goes into the Mediterranean diet, the only things that are left to be done are to try out these ravishing recipes and get on that path of redeeming your health! We hope you were inspired enough to follow this diet! Thank you again for downloading this e-book!

Part 2

Introduction

First of all, congratulations for making the move toward living a healthier lifestyle with the help of the Mediterranean Diet book! The Mediterranean Diet (also known as the Greek Diet or the Med. Diet) reflects a particular method of eating that is not only traditional to people in the Mediterranean but to others around the world as well, including celebrities. The foods you will eat on this diet are not only available in your local supermarket. It is also available at the farmer's market or even in your own backyard. In this book, we will cover everything from the history of the diet to the best foods to eat. Embracing the Mediterranean Diet and lifestyle is not just about making huge changes for the next few weeks, but is rather, about completely changing your relationship with foods. How you get them, how you prepare them and how you eat them.

Note: Don't forget to grab your FREE Bonus Report with the links at the end!

To start, there are seven fairly simple steps that will allow you to eat just like the Mediterranean's do:

1. Start to eat a lot of colorful vegetables. It does not really matter how. You can go for a simple plate of sliced or diced fresh tomatoes that have been drizzled with olive oil and crumbled feta cheese (low fat), spend hours crafting delicious salads with garlicky greens and delicious dressing or spend your time making fragrant soups and stews. Using vegetables, you can even make yourself some healthy pizzas or oven-roasted medleys that contain all of your favorite veggies with just a little olive oil for healthy fats. All vegetables are incredibly important keys to the freshest tastes and most delicious flavors of the Mediterranean Diet.

2. Put away the hamburger, eat some scallops. In all honesty, this is a pretty tasty trade off! If you like to eat or enjoy eating foods that have meats in them, then just use smaller amounts of leaner meat – small strips of chicken or sirloin mixed in a vegetable sauté will still give you a ton or flavor. Better yet, get yourself a nice plate of your favorite pasta accompanied by high quality diced prosciutto.

3. Enjoy those dairy products you love without any guilt. Unlike other diets, the Mediterranean Diet won't shame you for eating dairy! Eat Greek or plain yogurt with some berries for breakfast, and try smaller amounts of a variety of cheeses. Always try to go towards the non-fat or low-fat versions of your favorite dairy products.

4. Eat seafood at least twice a week, if not more. Once again, this is a tall order for people who really love foods. Fish such as haddock, tuna, herring, salmon, and sardines are some of the best meats for you because they are rich in omega-3 fatty acids. The same can also be said about many types of shellfish, including mussels, oysters, and clams! They have similar benefits to fish for the brain and the heart – just don't dunk them all in butter!

5. Cook a vegetarian meal (no meat or fish) at least one night a week. Though it might be difficult to do at first, building your meals and even your snacks around beans, whole grains, and vegetables will not only heighten the flavors with aromatic and tasty herbs and spices. It will also help you shrink your waistline. As you continue on the Med path, try to do this two nights per week or as a daylong activity.

6. Use (and enjoy) good fats. Include sources of healthy fats in all of your daily meals and snacks, especially in the forms of extra-virgin olive oil, nuts, peanuts, sunflower seeds, olives, and avocados. See later in this book for help on how to find and use the best EVOO!

7. If you have not yet made the switch to whole grains, do it now. Whole grains make up a HUGE part of the Med diet because they are naturally rich in many important nutrients that act to keep you on your feet and keep your body running. Cook with the traditional Mediterranean grains like bulgur, barley, farro and brown, black or red rice and favor products made with whole grain flour.

What is the Mediterranean Diet?

The Mediterranean Diet is a nutritional and lifestyle model that is based on the way those in the ancient Mediterranean (and to some extent, those who live there today) ate and lived their lives. It has more to do with nutrition, as it caters to the type of foods that they consume, the way their food is prepared, the way it is preserved (or not preserved, as the case may be) and the times at which they eat.

The Mediterranean Diet is rich in quality, safety, and cooking styles of food. The meals are almost always colorful, rich in spices, and much more frequent meals than those of us in the United States are prone to enjoy. The diet also leads to the overall health of the body and a general lack of metabolic diseases such as obesity, diabetes, hypertension, and many others. Though there is no proof behind this, there has also been a correlation between fewer mental health problems, learning disabilities and birth defects with the Mediterranean Diet.

Most importantly, this diet is critically important to the communities where it originated because of the sustainable development that is very important for all of the countries bordering on the Mediterranean Sea, and those that follow the lifestyle. It is critical to the economic and cultural systems within these countries because the food that is generally eaten can be grown, harvested, processed and sold throughout the region. The food then has the innate ability to inspire a sense of continuity and identity for local people as well as provide them with all that they will truly need for prosperity.

The diet is characterized by using a balance of foods that can be grown in the region including those foods that are rich in fiber (allow you to feel fuller longer), antioxidants (remove toxins from the body) and unsaturated (healthy) fats. Together, these create a healthy approach to eating animal fats and obtaining cholesterol. This diet also focuses on something called macros or macronutrients. In a typical Mediterranean Diet, the daily breakdown is simple:

55-60% Carbohydrates

80% of that is complex carbs like breads, pastas, rice, and anything made from flour

The rest is from fruits and vegetables that are locally grown with few preservatives

10-15% Proteins

60% of those proteins come from animals, focusing in on white meats, fish, and seafood

The rest comes from legumes and protein-rich plant-based foods and yogurts

25-30% Fats

Mostly comes from Olive Oil

The diet itself closely lines up with the nutritional standards that many Americans know. However, the sources of these percentages come from places we typically don't get them. Most Americas eat red meats that are virtually missing from the overall diet plan.

History of the Mediterranean Diet

The Mediterranean Diet traces its origins to a particular region of the world that is known as the Mediterranean Basin. Historians often refer to this area as "the cradle of society" because it is known as the starting place of modern life – from the way we perform politics to the way we eat. This civilization stretched from the valley of the Nile River. The East and West into the lands that were home to the Sumerians, Assyrians, Babylonians, and Persians along the Tigris and Euphrates Rivers. This region was home to some of the most powerful establishments in history like the Romans, the Phoenicians, and the Greeks, all of which rival our own systems today. These cultures effortlessly, for the most part, blended together cultures of different customs, languages, religions, and ways of thinking for the betterment of society. It was during these meetings that their eating habits came together into a melting pot of sorts, and the "Mediterranean Diet" was born.

Much of which foods came from which area is lost to history, but we do know that the eating habits of these people came from the Middle Ages and Roman tradition. The Greeks in particular considered breads, wines, and oils to be symbols of the prosperity and culture, bolstered by the trade and agricultural communities. They often fed on vegetables, cheese, fish, seafood and very little meat. In particular, they enjoyed leeks, lettuce, mallow, chicory, mushrooms, oysters and breads. The poorest in Rome, the slaves, survived mostly on bread and another staple of the diet, olives. Slaves in Rome would eat as many as half a pound of olives a month, as they were so plentiful. This also paved the path for olive oil.

As the Muslims grew in power, they impacted the diet by bringing in different plant species and specifically introducing them to the wealthier social classes. Some of what they introduced include rose water, oranges, lemons, almonds, sugar cane, rice, citrus, eggplant, spinach and spices, and the beloved pomegranate. Many Muslims also passed on their cooking and food preparation in a new culinary model.

However, as time changed, so did the diet that many in the Mediterranean enjoyed. One of the greatest historical events in terms of impact was the discovery of the Americas, particularly North America. These news lands and the people who lived there introduced potatoes, tomatoes, corn, peppers, chili, and a plethora of different types of beans. The tomato, in particular, is considered to be one the greatest food discoveries for the Mediterranean diet. Today, it is one of the primary symbols of the cuisine.

Bread, polenta, couscous, soups, paella, and pasta, all integral parts of the Mediterranean diet, all grew from the love of the exotic tomato. Much of the food one eats in the Mediterranean and while on the diet includes vegetables. Vegetables were key because they were easy to cook, were able to be eaten raw, supplemented meals, filled the poorer classes quickly, and added beauty to the plates that the cooks prepared. People particularly enjoyed making soups for the servants and the slaves with thin bases that used the "ends" of the vegetables that were prepared for the richer families. Sometimes these soups would contain meats, but that was not typical.

The "discovery" of the Mediterranean Diet and the health benefits it presents was actually documented by a scientist from America named Ancel Keys who studies at the University Of Minnesota School Of Power. He studied the diet for years and found that there was a correlation between cardiovascular disease and diet. He could not give a complete explanation at first but looked at the populations of different countries and the risk of death by cardiovascular disease. He found that towns full of the richest people in the world like New York City in the United States, as well as many other places within developed countries like the United States and throughout Europe had a higher risk of cardiovascular problems than those living in smaller, poorer towns and countries like those in southern Italy and the surrounding areas. He also found that those who had relatives that emigrated from Southern Italy were far less healthy overall than those who stayed.

When he found this correlation, he decided to dig deeper and created the "Seven Countries Study" which covered Finland, Holland, Italy, the United States, Greece, Japan, and Yugoslavia. He studied the relationship between nutrition, cardiovascular diseases and lifestyle choices. In this study, he proved scientifically the nutritional value of the Mediterranean diet and the Mediterranean lifestyle and its contribution to the health of the populations that adopted it. From this study, it emerged that the population who followed the more Mediterranean Diet had very low cholesterol in the blood, and therefore had healthy arteries and hearts. This led to better blood flow and mental clarity. This was mainly due to the daily diets (excluding holidays) and the use of olive oil, bread, pasta, vegetables, herbs, garlic, red onions and other foods of vegetable origin compared to a rather moderate use of meat.

Goods Fats v. Bad Fats

If it feels like the talk about fats is part of almost every diet - that's because it is. There are fats you need to have in your diet to keep everything moving, and there are fats you really want to limit to keep you moving. It would not do you any good to cut all fats from your diet. High-fat diets (like Atkins) have some pretty interesting problems as well. Simply put: your diet needs to have a healthy supply of HEALTHY fats to keep your body in tip-top shape. These fats provide the essential fatty acids you need to keep your skin soft, deliver fat-soluble vitamins to the rest of your body and provide you with energy for daily needs and exercise. Still, it's not always easy to see which fats are good and which fats are bad. Part of the Mediterranean Diet is to learn about how much fat you should eat, which fats are bad and will most likely clog your arteries (trans fats) and how omega-3 fatty acids (good fats) actually support overall heart health.

We have already covered how much fat you should have in a day on the Mediterranean Diet (as a refresher: 25-30%). The U.S. Department of Agriculture suggests that full sized adults should get about 20-35% of their calories from health fats. Even "low fat" diets suggest at least 10% - needless to say, they are important to weight loss.

Many Americans are eating much more fat in a day than they even realize. Some Americans are eating upwards of 40-50% of their daily calories from just high-fat foods. These foods generally taste "better" to the American palate and are more widely available to every person. They are also cheaper, easier to make, and require less preparation time.

It is so very easy for most people to overeat fats, even healthy fats, because they lurk in so many foods we love: French fries, processed foods, cakes, cookies, chocolate, ice cream, thick steaks, and cheese. Eating too much fat is a sure way to expand our waistlines and put unnecessary stress on our hearts. This fat then leads to inflammation which can lead to type 2 diabetes, certain forms of cancer and any type of heart disease.

Truth be told, all fats really do have about the same number of calories, so you cannot go from that alone. Choosing healthier fats just makes the food you eat better for your heart, it might not cut out things like breast cancer, colon cancer, knee and joint pain, and many other problems that plague those with higher BMIs.

Good Fats

For the easiest way to understand fats, there are two different groups: Saturated fats and unsaturated fats. Within each group of fats, there are many different types of fats.

The good guys are the unsaturated fats — these are the ones you want to stock up on. Unsaturated fats also include two other types of fats: polyunsaturated fatty acids and monounsaturated fats. Both of these types, when eaten in moderation and as part of an overall balanced diet, will actually help to lower cholesterol levels and reduce the risk of heart disease and other health problems. Polyunsaturated fats, found mostly in thing that you will use to cook, including vegetable oils, will actually help to lower both blood cholesterol levels and triglyceride levels -- especially when you use them as a substitute for those unhealthy saturated fats. One category of polyunsaturated fat is the ever famous omega-3 fatty acids, all of which have a very high potential heart-health benefits, and have gotten a lot of attention from not only the

Mediterranean Diet, but from other types of diets across the world.

Omega-3s are most often found in many types of fatty fish, including those that are frequently commercially available like salmon, trout, catfish, mackerel, as well as flaxseed and walnuts. These are the staples of the Mediterranean diet. It is those fish that contains the most effective, "long-chain" type of omega-3s that are the best building blocks for heart health. The Mediterranean Diet suggests getting at least three servings of these foods per week. You can use the plant sources like flaxseeds and walnuts, but they are not quite as good at decreasing cardiovascular diseases. Of course, don't even think about battering and deep frying your fish – that will take away any and all of the benefits! It is also suggested that you get these omega-3s from actual foods, not from supplements.

The other type of unsaturated fats that you will want to include in your diet is monounsaturated fats. These fats reduce the risk of heart disease in those who consume them. Once again, Mediterranean countries and those that follow the Mediterranean Diet will consume a lot of this type of fat, mostly in the form of olive oils. During the study of this type of diet, much of heart health of the citizens of those countries with the lowest levels of heart disease was attributed to the consumption of olive oil.

Monounsaturated fats are easier to identify by people who aren't aware of the different types of fats because they are typically liquid at room temperature (where they are usually stored by people) but solidify if refrigerated. These heart-healthy fats are typically a good source of the antioxidant vitamin E, a nutrient often lacking in North American diets. They can be found in olives, avocados, hazelnuts, almonds, Brazil nuts, cashews, sesame seeds, pumpkin seeds, olive, canola, and peanut oils.

Bad Fats

Now, when there are good guys, there also have to be bad guys. Bad fats are the ones that should be used sparingly by anyone who wants to live a healthy life. These fats are the saturated fats and the trans-fatty acids. Both of these can raise cholesterol levels to dangerous heights, clog arteries quickly, and increase the risk for heart disease in otherwise healthy people.

Saturated fats, a staple of most American diets, unfortunately, are found in most animal products especially processed ones, including, but not limited to, meat, poultry skin, high-fat dairy, and eggs. They can also be found in some types of vegetable fats that are liquid at room temperatures, such as coconut and palm oils. Once again, that does not mean that you have to eliminate those foods that you love completely from your diet. It just means that you might have to find a balance or find a way to only enjoy those things once a week or on special occasions. You should not deny yourself a juicy steak on your birthday, but don't do it every week.

Natural trans-fats are not the type of concern that is really addressed in the Mediterranean diet or by most doctors, especially if you choose low-fat dairy products and lean meats like chicken. The real worry in the American diet (and the diet in other developing countries) is the artificial trans-fats. They're used extensively in frying, baked goods, cookies, icings, crackers, packaged snack foods, microwave popcorn, and even in things that are marketed as being "healthier" like some margarines.

Most people, especially nutritionists and scientists, actually think that trans-fats, especially artificial trans-fats, are more dangerous to the human body than saturated fats are.

Research in this area has grown astronomically in the last few decades. It has shown that even consuming the slightest amount of artificial trans-fats on a regular basis can and will increase the risk for heart disease in otherwise healthy individuals because it increases the LDL or "bad" cholesterol and decreases the HDL or "good" cholesterol.

The American Heart Association (AHA) actually recommends restricting your consumption of trans fat to less than 2 grams per day and that number includes the naturally occurring trans-fats! The U.S. Dietary Guidelines, which has gone through many changes, has almost always recommend keeping trans-fats consumption as low as possible. However, most nutritionists would agree that eliminating all trans-fats is not going to save an otherwise unhealthy diet.

Which Fat Is This?

Most foods will contain a combination of different kinds of fats, but you should classify and determine which once you eat by using the dominant fat. Here are some lists that will allow you to make a more informed decision about the type of fat you are eating.

Saturated Fats / Trans Fatty Acids
- Butter
- Lard
- Meats and lunchmeats
- Poultry or poultry skin
- Coconut Products
- Palm Oil
- Palm Kernel
- Palm Oil
- Dairy Products (unless low fat or skim)
- Partially hydrogenated oils

Polyunsaturated Fats
- Corn Oil
- Fish Oil
- Soybean Oil and soy
- Safflower oil
- Sesame Oil
- Cottonseed oil
- Sunflower Oil
- Nuts
- Seeds
- Seed Oils

Monounsaturated Fats
- Canola Oil
- Almond Oil
- Walnut Oil
- Olive Oil
- Peanut Oil
- Avocados
- Black or Green Olives
- Peanut Butter

- Dehydrated Peanut Butter

Learning to Read Labels

The best way to learn and understand fats and to keep on top of the amount of fats in your diet is to start reading the labels on your foods. On the nutritional facts panel or chart, you will find all of the information you really need to make more healthy choices. In general, look for the foods that are low in the total amounts of fat – including saturated and trans-fat levels. Remember to keep in mind that a product that is marketed as low trans-fat or whose label boasts it is "trans-fat free" can actually have up to 0.5 grams of trans fats per serving -- and that can add up quickly if is it what you are cooking with for a large amount of your diet.

Here are just some extra tips that will allow you to reduce the total amount of fat in your diet and make sure the fats you consume are the healthy ones:

- Try to choose a diet that is rich in whole grains, fruits, and vegetables so you won't miss the sheer amount of food.
- Try to consume a vegetarian meal, with plenty of healthy beans, at least once a week.
- Select dairy products, if you must, that are skim or low-fat.
- Experiment with light and reduced-fat salad dressings until you can find one that you like.
- Replace fattier sauces like Alfredo, dressing and even some pasta sauces with vinegars, mustards, and lemon juice.
- When using fats, do so sparingly and after exhausting other options.
- Try to use unsaturated liquid oils, such as canola or olive, instead of butter or partially hydrogenated margarine.
- Try to limit your consumption of high-fat foods, such as processed foods,

fried foods, sweets and desserts to special occasional only.
- When cooking, substitute the lower-fat alternative (for example, low-fat milk products or low-fat cream cheese) whenever possible

The Science Behind the Best Olive Oils

Most people who are just starting out with the Mediterranean Diet will have to go out and buy their first official bottle of Olive Oil or Extra Virgin Olive Oil (affectionately known to some as EVOO). For others, you might want to reach for that old bottle that you've had for years – either way, you should probably just start with a new bottle. There are questions then on which is the best brand, the best region, or the best type to buy. Do you choose based on price? On labels? On which country it came from? Much like with buying high-quality wine, chocolate, or cheese, the science behind buying the best olive oils can take some time to acquire.

As olive oils have become more prevalent in American cuisine, we have been able to get more and more types of olive oil to line the shelves. We even make more olive oil in our country today than we ever have before! You will want to pay attention to quality, regulation, and taste when you are picking your oil.

Some Shopping Aisle Thoughts

When you are shopping, there are some things you should definitely be on the lookout for when it comes to your olive oil purchase. You will want to look for a label that tells you that the olives have been cold pressed. This means that there was no type of heat used in the pressing or crushing process, meaning that the olive's chemistry was kept intact, ensuring the highest amount of nutrients. For the olive oil to give you the most benefits, it will need to be as natural as possible.

Storage

Another reason that you will want to avoid heat, as well as light and oxygen is because it can cause the olive oil to go back or just not taste as good. You will want to look for olive oil that is stored in thick, dark green glass packaging that is away from the lights. Do not take any olive oils that are sitting in direct sunlight, and do not purchase any olive oils that are in plastic containers. Continue this practice when you take the product home, store it in a cool, dark place at home, or wrap the bottle in aluminum foil to shield it from further sunlight. Do not store near any heat sources like on top of the stove or oven or in adjacent cabinets.

Color

While many people who are new to olive oil will think that the green olive oil must be richer in flavors and nutrients than yellow olive oil, this is not the case at all. In fact, the color of the actual olive oil really indicates nothing at all about the way it tastes or what it does for your body. It's all about the way the oil tastes, feels and lingers in your mouth, the way it interacts with other foods and the way it was crushed. Remember that light-colored oils can be high quality, as well as darker oils. In fact, some companies that know about this rumor have taken advantage of this myth by adding leaves to the olive crush, which increases chlorophyll and achieves a darker green color, while upping the price and not really doing too much for you.

Light Olive Oil v Regular Olive Oil

There is no such thing as a "light" or "diet" extra virgin olive oil or olive oil. If you see these, check the ingredients and see if you are really getting olive oil. They do not exist, and anyone who tries to sell you a product like this will probably also sell you a beach house in Alaska! A lighter color, once again for emphasis, absolutely does not mean that the olive oil is any lower in calories. In fact, purchasing anything that says it is "light" has almost surely been chemically (i.e. processed so not that great for you) treated to minimize strong smells and tastes that actually suggests an inferior oil.

Common Questions about Olive Oils

Aren't all types and brands of olive oils more or less the same exact thing?

If you've read this far into the book, you know that the answer is absolutely no. Variations in fruit intensity that you can find are delicate, medium and robust. Then there is always the supermarket problem and the pitfall of mislabeled qualities. If the label says "extra virgin olive oil" or "pure olive oil" (the highest qualities available on the market), don't believe it even a little bit until you have done some poking around on the internet. There is a lot of inferior oil that sometimes gets used, usually called "virgin" oil or "pomace" oil that gets a top-quality label when in reality it is actually a lesser quality oil used to drive up prices. Extra virgin olive oil should have absolutely no defects at all– there should be no bad smells nor should it have any bad or bitter tastes and it needs to be balanced with a certain amount of pungency or spiciness in the throat.

How do I differentiate between types and intensities?

Unfortunately, this is not an easy thing to do and it takes practice. Try to think of it as a spice that can be added to food. Start out by buying a brand we recommend and then experiment with it. Food pairings are very subjective—you might like delicate oil on a salad or even a citrus oil. And it's amazing how an oil's flavor can change when combined with certain foods.

When you are looking, you will more likely see three different general categories of olive oils: delicate oils, medium oils, and robust oils. You can also find flavored oils, but that probably isn't your best bet. Furthermore, most producers will not differentiate for you on the bottle. There are some ways you can tell, especially if your bottle tells you which olives were used:

Delicate oil (made from Arbequina, Leccino, Sevillano, Taggiasca olives) is usually the choice of most cooks that want a garnish for fish. This is a much lighter type of oil, and you would not want to drown out a delicate, mild white fish with an overpowering oil.

Medium-intensity oil (Ascolana, Manzanillo, Mission olives) will mostly go well as a base for homemade salad dressing or to add additional flavor to grilled vegetables and poultry.

Robust oil (Arbosana, Frantoio, Picholine olives) is the best option (in general, not on the Mediterranean diet) to drizzle over steak with a spritz of lemon.

Is there a big health or Mediterranean Diet difference between using cooked (or heated) and uncooked olive oil?

Uncooked olive oil is going to be the much healthier option when compared to cooked olive oil. When you apply heat, a chemical change occurs at its smoking point. It essentially begins to consume itself through burning and cuts the nutrients nearly in half. Plus, using the raw oil will help you to maintain its great, pure flavor while heating or cooking and adding in too many other ingredients may change the flavor of the cooked oil, making it less appetizing. The best way to use oil for cooking is to just use the minimum amount needed to complete the job and then go ahead garnish the dish with oil from the bottle (depending on how much you need to complete your macros or servings) just before serving.

Is unfiltered olive oil a better, healthier choice when trying to maintain a Mediterranean Diet?

Unfiltered olive oil, extra virgin olive oil or pure olive oil - in the end, it doesn't really matter. Unfiltered olive oil does not go through a filter and tends to have a slight cloudiness to it. Unfiltered olive oil also has a marginally higher polyphenol (antioxidant) content and a slightly longer shelf life (only slightly, but if you follow the Mediterranean Diet, that really won't matter). At the end of the day, though, it just comes down to your personal preference.

Can I enjoy flavored oils (citrus, truffle) while on the Mediterranean Diet?

In short, yes. Many of the flavored oils will have just about the same issue as extra virgin olive oils do in terms of evaluating quality. A person who is on the Mediterranean Diet can use citrus flavored oils or, instead, experiment with adding juice or zest directly to the dish. But think. How can a mandarin olive oil enhance a well-prepared entrée? Or how can a high-quality lemon olive oil accent fish? Truffle oil (or truffle butter as some call it, depending on what you're making) is the perfect way to add that beloved truffle flavor without having to go on a hunt and pay for the real thing (especially because quality, fresh truffles are only available a couple times a year). It is important, however, to choose a trusted brand when it comes to flavored oils and butters, as they can be enhanced chemically.

Should I use extra virgin olive oil for frying if I want to?

Well, frying anything is hardly part of the Mediterranean Diet. In the end, it really depends on what and how you are going to fry. Generally the answer without thinking about your diet is "yes." Most of the alternative and inferior oils that claim to be healthier for frying have actually been put through a chemical treatment to strip obvious defects and produce a neutral flavor. Processing is always a bad idea. Of course, if you are frying and calories aren't really a problem, extra virgin olive oil has a great taste that will most likely complement whatever you're frying.

Still Confused? Try a Taste Test!

Are you still a little confused about trying out olive oil brands? Here is a system that will help you choose between a few different ones if you have a taste test:

Pour a bit of your chosen oil into a small glass, you might want to start with the lightest, just for your own records. Warm the liquid up by moving the class around in your hands so that the aroma and flavor of the oils are magnified.

Sip a very small amount of the oil into your mouth and make short sucking sounds along your lower jaw line toward the back of your mouth. You will want to feel and taste the oil as it travel throughout your mouth and to your taste buds.

Close your mouth while holding the oil and breathe out of your nose to allow your nasal cavity to process the smells and the taste of the oil.

Swallow just a very small amount to understand and the pungency of the oil in your throat.
Spit out the rest into a separate bowl.

If there is any sign of a waxy residue in your mouth or any astringency (drying of mouth), these are indicators of rancidity and that means that you can cross that off of your list.

Before you go on to try any other type of oil (or really any other type of food), cleanse your palate with water and slices of green apple.

Mediterranean Foods

There is always some confusion when it comes to what someone can and cannot eat while they are on the Mediterranean Diet.

Some of the dietary data from the parts of the Mediterranean has given many different nutritionists and scientists the best possible data about what foods people should be eating and what foods they should try to avoid in general. The healthfulness of this particular eating pattern isn't just something new like some of the newer diet fads that are around. In fact, this particular method is proven by more than 50 years of research as well as hundreds of years of civilization research focusing in on medical documents. The basics of the Mediterranean Diet plan include the following rules and regulations on your diet:

- A fairly high percentage of the foods that you will eat on this plan come from plant sources. These include fruits and vegetables, some potatoes, breads, especially grainy breads, beans, some nuts, and seeds.

- There is also a large amount of emphasis on minimally processed and seasonally fresh foods, when they are available. To do this, focus in on foods that are grown locally and attend farmer's markets and local farmer stands. Doing this will ensure the highest amount of nutrients from the foods.

- Olive oil absolutely must be the principal fat that you consume. It should act as a replacement for all of the other fats and oils in your diet, including any margarine and butter.

- Your total fat should range from less than 25 percent of your daily calorie usage to over 35 percent of the energy, with saturated fat being absolutely no more than 7 to 8 percent.

- You should try to work in daily consumption of low to moderate amounts of cheese and yogurt that is low fat or non-fat.
- You should aim to get in two servings of fish or poultry in a week. You can also use up to 7 eggs per week total, including in baking and cooking. Remember that fish tends to be favored over poultry.
- Fresh fruits should make up the majority of your desserts or "sweets." Sweets that have a substantial amount of sugar, honey, fake sweeteners and saturated fat should not be consumed more than 1-2 times per week.
- Remember that you are allowed to eat red meat a few times per month. Research has shown that people who are used to red meat and then completely restrict it are more likely to fail on the Mediterranean Diet.
- Remember that while most weight loss and health is about 80% based on your diet, you still need to get inappropriate

amounts of exercise and physical activity.

For Men

For some guys, it may not seem very manly, but in actuality, the Mediterranean Diet is one of the best possible ways for men of all ages, not only live longer and healthier lives, but also the ability to eat well. It will make you look like you know your way around the kitchen, which is one of the sexiest things a man can do. Plus it doesn't hurt that you will keep fit and save some money at the same time. The biggest bonus for most men? Heart disease is the #1 cause death for otherwise healthy American men. This means that it is critical for you to know and consume foods that are heart healthy. If you already know them, then you need to know how to include them in a daily meals.

The Mediterranean Diet is ONE of the Manliest Diets

With this diet, you will eat large portions of food, leaving you satisfied and reducing the cravings for snacks. The Mediterranean Diet is based upon age-old practices that everyone from doctors to warriors ate – making it extremely nourishing and filling. This is because you will have plenty of protein and healthy fats to fill yourself with. There no bird food here, with foods such as olive oil, seafood, eggs, and Greek yogurt filling your stomach. Plus you won't feel like you are restricting yourself because you have fiber-rich whole grains that will keep you feeling pleasantly full and satisfied for hours without feeling like you are eating the same things over and over again. Oh, and these foods also help lower cholesterol and keep arteries clear.

The Mediterranean Diet is unlike many other diets because it includes plenty of whole foods, meals, and recipes that have the big flavors, spices, and soups that men crave and love: pasta and rice, hearty bean soups and stews, as well as modest servings of lean red meat, with plenty of opportunity to add herbs and spices for extra zing. All of these foods add up you learning your way around the kitchen. Women tend to eat lighter meals than men do anyway, so learning how to cook these foods will certainly impress the woman in your life. No one wants a man that can just make grilled cheese and Ramen Noodles!

Living a Mediterranean way will also encourage you to start liking the foods that are really good for you. You will have vegetables in ways you have never had them before, and they may even change your mind about things like chicory or prunes. Studies have shown that men who consistently eat a diet that is rich in colorful vegetables, fish, nuts, and legumes, have a higher level of protection against certain kinds of cancers, including colon and testicular cancers. As a bonus, they may also help reduce periodontal diseases, meaning you can keep your teeth!

For those of you that are getting older, men tend to put weight on around their waists as they start getting up there in age and their metabolism slows down. Following the Mediterranean Diet and following it strictly, can actually slow down your weight gain and speed up the slowing metabolism that is normally observed as men get over a certain age. Including more plant-based foods like vegetables, fruits, and legumes while still being cognizant of maintaining a healthy unsaturated: saturated fat ratio can (and will!) have positive effects on your lower abdominal obesity (below your belly button) and reduce the risk of developing coronary heart disease.

Do you find yourself having brain fog about important dates of figures? Consuming foods that follow the Mediterranean Diet, such as olive oil, whole grains, fish, healthy fats, and fruits protect you from the brain fog and confusion that comes aging brains. All of these problems come from damage linked to cognitive problems and helps lower the risk of Alzheimer's, Dementia, and other memory problems.

Finally, if all of that didn't convince you to follow this diet plan, consider the fact that men who follow the Mediterranean diet are less likely to suffer from erectile dysfunction and have more stamina and strength in the bedroom.

For Women

Women are more likely to try a diet when it comes out than men are. However, a woman's body chemistry makes almost every "fad" diet seem like a failure. The Mediterranean Diet is different because it really isn't a diet at all, it's a healthy way of eating that can transform you – inside and out. It gives you a longer life and lowers your risk of diseases that kill more women each year than anything else. Not only that, but the Mediterranean Diet seems to go along with the foods that women naturally love.

Heart health is just one problem that women face as they age – osteoporosis hinders the lives of thousands of women each and every year, and the Mediterranean Diet has led to some of the strongest and toughest women around. These foods are good for your bones! You will be able to choose from food sources that not only contain the important nutrients that you need for health, but it will also allow you to get into the habit of eating a wide variety of colorful foods every day. The Mediterranean Diet is far more effective when it comes to the way a woman's body works and loses weight. Say goodbye to those crash diets, continuous workouts or skipping or scrimping on meals for weight maintenance and healthy bodies.

Mediterranean Ingredients

Here are some important reasons as to why women should incorporate various Mediterranean ingredients into their diets:

The variety of greens will keep you regular and feeling great. You don't just have a few to choose from, you can pick from anything and make a delicious salad or a green smoothie. These options include greens, cucumbers, avocados, sprouts, peppers, carrots, celery, broccoli, and summer squash. The possibilities are endless with these foods – eat them raw, steam them, mix them into an omelet, or make them into a stir-fry! These foods will also help with stopping osteoporosis right in its tracks. Calcium rich foods like Greek yogurt, Brussel sprouts, collard greens, spinach, broccoli, kale, and beans will strengthen you bones and give you back that density.

Another benefit of following along with the Mediterranean Diet is the sheer amount of potassium that your diet will include. The Mediterranean Diet includes foods like potatoes, greens, legumes, and probably a new one for you, winter squash that all give your body the nutrients that encourage the development of muscles and lower blood pressure, which are especially important to women.

Especially during "that time of the month," women need to incorporate more iron-rich foods into their diets. These are very easy to put into your meal plan as lentils, spinach, almonds, lean red meat and dark meat poultry are good sources of iron. These are also great options for people who have anemia. Iron is also necessary to keep your heart healthy, which is the main reason the Mediterranean Diet works on all of these levels. You won't even have to make many changes to your current diet to get these heart-healthy benefits. Start with whole grains in your morning cereal or oatmeal, add some berries and then get some fiber so that you can stay satisfied. What's the best part? Those foods will flush the toxins out of your body and will keep your arteries clear. Mix it up the next day and include some Greek yogurt!

Many women think that fat in their foods automatically equals fat on their waists, butts, hips, thighs, or arms. However, that is not the case either – you should NOT avoid fats. Healthy fats, as you have learned, reduce your risk of heart disease, build up the shine in your hair, keep your skin clear, and make your fingernails hard. What is the point of being super skinny if the rest of you is falling apart? Healthy fats will also be able to keep you feel fuller for a longer time after you have a meal, reducing your cravings and lessening those snack attacks that lead to you bingeing on ice cream at midnight. Plus, "good" fat also help your body during other important times, as it promotes a healthy pregnancy, makes for an easier labor and is important for your baby's developing brain.

Most Important Ingredients from the Mediterranean Diet for Women

These four foods are the most important ones for women to incorporate into their diets. While your diet needs to be balanced, focus on moving these into your kitchen as soon as possible:

Olive Oil or EVOO is rich in those good fats that we just mentioned, plus it adds a delicate flavoring and savory feeling to just about everything you eat.

Fish is a super secret for celebrities, models, and female athletes alike. The best fish for women is Salmon, which is especially rich in those omega-3 fatty acids that you need for beauty and for your body. If you can't start with salmon because you don't like the fishy taste, consider wading in gently with seafood like scallops, shrimp, or lobster.

Nuts and peanuts are not always a popular choice for women, for some reason. However, keeping a can or pack of nuts in your drawer at work will stop you from taking a trip to the vending machine. If you are looking for some crunch for your yogurt or salad, consider adding them to the top for an additional flavor that adds healthy fats. Remember that a serving of nuts like almonds or hazelnuts is about ¼ cup!

Finally, add olives to your salads, sandwiches, and just as a snack for at night. They are low calorie, fulfill your need for salty foods while still having the monounsaturated fats, essential fatty acids, and natural antioxidants that you need to follow the Mediterranean Diet.

Conclusion

It is my sincere hope that you might have liked all the recipes which have been mentioned in the book and once again thank you for getting this book and experimenting with the recipes.

About The Author

Sara Shirley is born with the vision to promote *Mediterranean diet* among the masses. The author has written several research papers on the topic. He has served as an instructor promoting various cultural arts in University of San Francisco. He is currently living with his spouse in Texas.

www.ingramcontent.com/pod-product-compliance
Lightning Source LLC
LaVergne TN
LVHW020424080526
838202LV00055B/5031